ONE BODY—
ONE LIFE

"Where there is life, there is hope.
Live life more abundantly".

ONE BODY—
ONE LIFE

Health Screening
   Disease Prevention
      Personal Health Record
         Leading Causes of Death

DR. YAN PERUMAL

MBCHB, M.MED (Family Medicine), FRACGP, CIME (ABIME)
- **Family Physician**
- **Certified Independent Medical Examiner (American Board)**

To order additional copies of this book, contact:
Xlibris LLC
1-800-455-039
www.xlibris.com.au
Orders@xlibris.com.au
503343

CONTENTS

Dedication

This book is dedicated to my late parents. Due to extreme poverty, neither enjoyed the privilege of any formal education. Yet they imparted knowledge and wisdom far beyond the borders of academic learning .The heritage they left behind has become a legacy to my siblings and I, the extended family, and the wider community. We will forever be grateful.

Acknowledgments

I thank my wife, Dr Moira Perumal, for her love, support and contribution throughout this venture.

I feel humbled that the following leading academic medical professionals had agreed to read and provide invaluable expert advice:

Professor M.H. Cassimjee, Nelson Mandela School of Medicine, University of Kwa-Zulu Natal, Durban, South Africa.

and

Dr Sanne Kreijkamp-Kaspers, Senior Research Fellow, School of Medicine, University of Queensland, Australia

I acknowledge the assistance of several individuals representing various professions and walks of life, who sacrificed much of their valuable time to read, advise corrections and make useful comments regarding the content and structure of the book.

I am grateful to the rest of my family and friends for their encouragement through this journey.

I am thankful for insights and knowledge I derived from all my teachers across the globe, extending over several decades.

I appreciate my colleagues in medical practice with whom I have shared experiences over the years for our mutual benefit. I acknowledge them as the ultimate gatekeeper's of a patient's wellbeing.

FOREWORD

A handbook of this nature has been long overdue. The primary focus of the book is on Health promotion and Health screening. I expect it to generate much interest amongst the lay public in general. The handbook is an easy to read document and user friendly. The language flows easily and can be understood by people in both developed and developing countries, anywhere in the world. The book sends a clear message that while the health professional can care for the patient, the individual patient is still ultimately responsible for his or her own health. Patients are advised to take cognisance of the issues raised and the importance of forging a partnership with their Family Practitioner.

The book highlights the common medical problems plaguing mankind. It importantly addresses ways and methods of identifying problems early so as to prevent end stage disasters. This is perhaps the core strength of this handbook. The contents have been dealt with in sufficient depth, and provide useful websites and references, should a patient decide to seek further information.

I believe this handbook has international value, providing a well-researched, comprehensive, yet easily readable and informative document which has been long overdue.

It has been my privilege and honour to have had the opportunity to review this excellent manuscript.

Professor M.H.Cassimjee

LLMRCP, LLMRCS (Ireland), M.Med (Family Medicine), MFGP (SA), FCFP (SA), B.Med Science Hons. (Pharmacology), Dip. Health Services Management.

- Honorary Professor, Department of Family Medicine, Nelson Mandela School of Medicine, Durban, South Africa.
- Technical Advisor-World Health Organisation (Special projects)
- Secretary General of African Gulf Society of Sexual Medicine

10th July 2013

So much effort and money is wasted worldwide by managing health problems that could have been prevented. We have a habit of fixing things only when they are broken. What if we changed that and started looking after them and prevent them from breaking in the first place?

Dr Yan Perumal has written this concise, practical book to help us understand disease prevention. By observing the advice offered in this book we can make changes to care for our bodies in the best possible way. In so doing we will make a positive difference to our own lives, those of our families and the community as a whole.

Dr Sanne Kreijkamp-Kaspers

MD (Netherlands), PhD, FRACGP (Australia), MSc.

Senior Research Fellow

Discipline of General Practice, School of Medicine

University of Queensland

Australia.

16th July 2013

CHAPTER 1

Introduction

In recent years the focus of attention in healthcare worldwide has shifted from the emphasis on curing diseases to preventing them if possible. A large financial burden goes hand in hand with the cost of treating preventable diseases. A significant portion of budgets in virtually every country is consumed by managing preventable diseases. Sadly this financial cost could be considered a wasteful loss of useful resources which could be used for other more pressing human issues worldwide. Poverty, lack of resources, poor education and political issues all combine, resulting in negative and sometimes tragic health outcomes.

This book attempts, in an elementary way, to uncover a few basic concepts and guidelines to improving your health and help prevent disease. It is by no means intended to be a complete exposition of all the health issues of relevance. It cannot be emphasized enough that the most important guardians and guides to your healthcare is your family doctor and other health care providers. Ultimately they will be your most useful resources in preserving and promoting your health. It must be noted that protocols may vary from one country to another, in addition to changing over time. Hence it is vital that you keep updated with recent developments through your treating doctor.

I trust that this handbook will serve to stimulate thoughts about exploring issues more carefully around your health in the future. After all, your body and it's health, is your most valued asset. The better you care for it, the better your quality of life will be, and hopefully your lifespan. One may draw a simple parallel with the way we care for our other assets, for example, the regular servicing of our motor vehicles. How much more should this principle apply to the care of our personal health?

We have only "One Body and One Life". May we nurture it with the best possible care. In so doing, we will enjoy this one precious life to the maximum extent.

CHAPTER 2

Health Screening

Screening is a process of identifying disease in healthy people who have no symptoms. They may be individuals who are at increased risk of a disease or condition. These individuals can be offered information, further tests and appropriate treatment if needed. Health screening tests are conducted as a preventative measure.

High risk individuals are those who have risk factors that are likely to predispose them to impending disease. It should be noted that there is no universal agreement as to which tests should be performed for health screening and when they should be performed. Individual doctors or insurers may have their own protocols for health screening tests. What follows, then, are common recommendations. Individuals should consult their doctors and insurers for information specific to their needs. Frequently, data from health screenings give scientists a way of measuring disease trends and the success of early treatment. One is able to remove or reduce risks, arrive at an early diagnosis, commence treatment early and limit complications.

Disease prevention types fall into 3 categories:

1. Primary prevention.

This is prevention of diseases or disorders in the general population by encouraging community wide measures such as good nutritional status, physical fitness, immunisation and making the environment safe. Primary prevention maintains good health and reduces the likelihood of disease occurring.

2. Secondary prevention

This type aims at detecting early stages of the disease before symptoms occur, and the prompt and effective intervention to prevent disease progression.

3. Tertiary prevention

This type relates to prevention or minimisation of complications or disability associated with established disease. Preventative measures are part of the treatment or management of the target disease or condition.

Since the intensification of screening overall mortality has decreased worldwide. In particular, improvements have been noted with regards to congenital abnormalities, heart attacks, strokes, diabetes related complications, most infectious diseases, cancers of the skin, lung, stomach, colon, cervix and breast.

Your family doctor is ideally placed to undertake your health promotion and disease prevention. You should ensure your doctor has full knowledge of your personal and family health history. Your doctor can act as co-ordinator of preventative health measures.

Purposes for Health Screening

A periodic visit to your doctor can help you:

- Screen for potential underlying health problems.
- Assess your risk for future health problems.
- Treat current medical conditions.
- Update relevant vaccinations.
- Maintain a healthy doctor-patient relationship in the event of an illness arising in the future.

CHAPTER 3

Health Promotion

A periodic health check is a crucial part of ongoing wellbeing. Regular health examinations and tests can help find problems before they start. The specific examinations and screening you need will depend on your sex, age, health and family history, and your personal lifestyle choices. Many factors can affect your health. Some you cannot control, such as your genetic makeup or your age. But you can make changes to your lifestyle. By taking steps towards healthy living, you can help reduce your risk of heart disease, some cancers, stroke and other serious diseases. It is valuable to see your doctor for periodic health checks and take an active interest in your own healthcare. Lifestyle factors which influence health and disease are discussed next.

Healthy Eating and Weight

Calories are a measure of how much energy food or drinks contain. The amount of energy you need will depend on your age, sex, how active you are and your size (body mass index). Other factors can affect how much of calories you burn, for example, some hormones, medications or illness. An average man needs around 2500 calories a day, and an average woman needs around 2000 calories a day.

The advice is to eat a variety of healthy foods, limit calories to daily requirements, and limit saturated fats. The following is a general guide to a healthy eating pattern:

1. Eat sparingly:
    Fatty red meats, processed meats, white rice, white bread, pasta, fried potatoes, sugary drinks and sweets, salt and alcohol.
2. Eat in moderation:
    Dairy products, lean meats, poultry, fish, and eggs.
3. Eat freely:
    Vegetables, fruit, lentils, grains, beans, nuts (unsalted), whole wheat pasta and oats

Body mass index (BMI) and Waist to Hip Ratio are useful tools to calculate and monitor weight.

Definition of Body Mass Index: Weight (kg) divided by Height (metres) squared.

	Body Mass Index (BMI)
Healthy range	18.5-24.9
Underweight	less than 18.5
Overweight	25.0-29.9
Obese	30+

The desired Waist to Hip ratio measured in centimetres is as follows:

Men: 1.0 or lower

Women:-0.8 or lower

Obesity, in particular abdominal fat, is an important risk factor for heart disease, high blood pressure, diabetes and strokes, among other health issues.

Alcohol

The best overall health advice is not to drink alcohol. No one is able to predict the possibility of who could become dependent on alcohol to a point of abuse. Excessive alcohol usage can cause damage to multiple organs, decreasing the quality of life, increasing the risk of accidental and suicidal deaths, as well as reducing lifespan. In addition there are negative consequences in terms of social and family life, and legal implications.

If you are drinking alcohol, note that most guidelines advise limiting alcohol intake to no more than 2-3 standard drinks per day. Women who are pregnant or breastfeeding should not drink alcohol. Do not drink and drive. One should observe at least 2 alcohol free days per week.

One standard drink is defined as (approximately):

Percentage of alcohol	Volume
Wine (13%)	100 ml
Beer	
Full strength (4.8%)	285 ml
Mid strength (3.5%)	375 ml
Low strength (2.7%)	425 ml
Spirits:	
High strength (40%)	30ml nip
Full strength (5%)	
(ready to drink)	275 ml
High strength (7%)	
(ready to drink)	185 ml

A questionnaire called AUDIT (alcohol use disorders identification test) can be used to assist in diagnosing the possibility of problem drinking. The following are warning signs that you may have a problem of alcohol abuse:

- You, your family or friends are concerned about your level of alcohol intake.
- You are regularly drinking more than the limits suggested earlier.
- You are unable to stop drinking once you have started.
- You need a first drink in the morning.
- You feel guilty or remorseful after drinking.
- You injured yourself or someone else after drinking.

If some of the above apply to you, it is advised you seek medical help. You will be directed to organisations for advice and support.

Exercise

It is advised that one is physically active. Regular exercise is a critical part of staying healthy. People who are active feel better and live longer. The American Heart Association recommends that you do moderate exercise at least 150 minutes a week (around 30-40 minutes, 4 to 5 time a week) or 75 minutes (around 20 minutes, 3-4 times a week) of vigorous exercise. Adopt simple routines such as climbing stairs instead of taking the elevator, walking or cycling instead of driving the car, regularly taking your dog for a walk.

Recreational activities, such as playing sport, dancing or hobbies which require physical effort, are beneficial for both physical and mental wellbeing. No one is too young or too old to exercise. If you suffer any medical conditions, speak to you doctor about the appropriate program for you. An exercise physiologist can design an exercise program which will be safe for you. Stop exercising if you experience any worrying symptoms, such as chest pain, palpitations, unusual shortness of breath or dizziness. If the symptoms persist for more than a few minutes you should seek prompt medical attention. There is a saying that goes "use it or lose it". Lack of exercise is one of the factors in either the development of, or difficulty in controlling diseases such as heart disease, high blood pressure and diabetes.

Exercise can:

- Help control weight
- Combat heart disease, diabetes and high blood pressure
- Improve mood
- Boost energy
- Promote better sleep
- Improve bone health and prevent or delay osteoporosis
- Decrease depression and memory loss
- Improve sex life

Smoking

Smoking related diseases result in over 5 million deaths per year worldwide. This equates to around twenty percent of all deaths. The advice is not to commence smoking, or if you are smoking at present, seriously consider quitting. Seek medical advice to help you quit.

Tobacco is one of the leading preventable causes of death and disease worldwide. It is estimated that persistent smoking kills around half of tobacco users. Smoking around your family increases their risk of various diseases, including repeated chest infections and heart attacks by around 25%, among others. On average, smokers die around 10 years younger than non-smokers. Smoking is implicated in a vast range of morbidities in virtually every system in your body, affecting your quality of life, and resulting in premature deaths. Smoking causes an estimated 80-90% of all Lung cancer and chronic lung disease deaths. In addition smoking is implicated as a cause in a variety of other Cancers. More deaths are caused by smoking than by HIV/AIDS or motor vehicle accidents worldwide. It increases the incidence of Heart attacks and Strokes by 3-4 times that of non-smokers. A variety of abnormalities may occur in unborn babies of pregnant mothers who smoke.

Large sums of money, which could be used for other more important personal and family needs, such as food, clothing, accommodation, education and health maintenance are spent by smokers on tobacco products. Governments around the world spend exorbitant sums of tax payer funds on the treatment of smoking related illnesses. The good news is that after just one year of ceasing smoking your risk of heart disease is halved. It is advised that you talk to your doctor about various support mechanisms, counselling, nicotine replacement products and prescription medications which can help you quit.

Sleep

Adequate sleep plays an important role in both physical and mental wellbeing. Various physical and psychological conditions can interfere with normal sleep pattern. Sleep apnoea is a condition where a person experiences irregular breathing while asleep, excessive snoring, and excessive sleepiness during the day. The causes of sleep apnoea include obesity, smoking, excess alcohol intake, some drugs and abnormal jaw structure. Sleep apnoea can result in heart attacks, strokes, high blood pressure and irregular heart beat. If you find that you fall off to sleep easily while performing some of the following activities it is advised that you seek medical attention:

- Sitting and reading or watching television
- Sitting inactive in a theatre or meeting
- Sitting as a passenger in a car for an hour without a break, or after a few minutes of stopping at traffic lights
- Resting in the afternoon after lunch without alcohol
- Sitting and talking to someone

A sleep test (polysomnography) is performed by a specialist in sleep disorders to confirm a diagnosis of sleep apnoea.

The following are some suggestions to experience adequate sleep. This is annotated as "sleep hygiene".

- Do not oversleep
- Avoid lying in bed for long periods if you are unable to fall off to sleep. Rather get out of bed and engage in some physical or mental activity till you feel tired and are ready to sleep.
- Wake up at a regular time.
- Avoid bright lights.
- Avoid heavy meals in the evening.
- Avoid caffeine in the late afternoon or evening.
- Reduce alcohol intake and avoid smoking.
- Have a warm bath or shower before going to sleep.
- Sleep on a comfortable mattress and pillow.
- Sleep in a quiet, dark room.
- Perform regular exercise.

Sleep apnoea is managed by weight loss, mouth devices, the use of a C-Pap machine and occasionally surgery.

Spirituality and Health

Some research conducted by reputable institutions in different parts of the world has confirmed that religious involvement and spirituality are associated with better physical health, mental health, longevity, and overall quality of life. A study in the United States of America has reported that a voluntary organisation which was spiritually based recorded up to 70% success with drug addiction rehabilitation, as compared to a success rate of 15% with government funded programs.

CHAPTER 4

An overview of some Common Medical Conditions causing Death

Hypertension (High Blood Pressure)

It is estimated that around one third of adults above 25 years old suffer from high blood pressure worldwide. In 2011 around 8 million people worldwide died of complications of high blood pressure.

Normal blood pressure is 120/80 mmHg. Persistent blood pressure of 140/90 and above can be regarded as high blood pressure, and medical attention should be sought. In between these readings it is advised to monitor the blood pressure at around 3 monthly intervals.

The cause of high blood pressure is unknown in most cases.

This is called Essential Hypertension.

The risk is higher if you:

- have a family history of high blood pressure
- are of African/Caribbean origin
- are of the Indian Subcontinent origin

High blood pressure may be influenced by other factors such as:

- Obesity
- Excessive salt in the diet

- Alcohol overuse
- Smoking
- Diabetes
- Lack of exercise
- Kidney disease
- Some medications
- Endocrine (chemical) conditions

Consequences of untreated High blood pressure include:

- Heart attack and heart failure
- Stroke and brain damage
- Kidney damage
- Blood vessel damage
- Pregnancy complications
- Eye and vision complications

Prevention or reduction of high blood pressure can be achieved by:

- Avoiding smoking
- Reducing alcohol intake
- Eating a healthy diet as outlined previously.
- Exercising regularly (30-45 minutes daily on most days)
- Maintaining your ideal weight
- Reducing chronic stress
- Controlling Diabetes
- Using Blood pressure reducing medications if needed

High Cholesterol /Fats

Cholesterol is a fat chemical. A certain amount of cholesterol is needed to stay healthy.

There is good Cholesterol (HDL Cholesterol), and bad fats (LDL Cholesterol and Triglycerides).

High Cholesterol can exist as a result of:

- Heredity
- Obesity or unhealthy diet
- Alcohol overuse
- Some kidney, thyroid and liver disorders

Persistently high total and LDL cholesterol may result in:

- Heart attack
- Stroke
- Blood clots/Blocked blood vessels

The risk of the above complications increase with Smoking, Obesity, Alcohol overuse, and poorly controlled Hypertension and Diabetes.

Guidelines for Lipid levels are as follows (slight variations exist between different countries):

Total cholesterol: around 5.0 mmol/l

LDL (undesirable): around 2.5 mmol/l

Triglycerides(undesirable): less than 2.0 mmol/l

HDL (desirable): above 1.0 mmol/l

Individuals with risk factors for cardiovascular disease (heart attacks, strokes) need to reach better targets.

Heart Attacks

In 2011 around 7 million people died of heart attacks worldwide, making it the leading cause of death.

A Heart attack is caused by an interruption of blood supply to a portion of heart muscle. It is the leading cause of death in high income earning countries.

Conditions increasing the risk of a heart attack include:

- High blood pressure
- Smoking
- High cholesterol (LDL cholesterol and triglycerides), and low HDL cholesterol
- Diabetes
- Obesity
- Alcohol abuse
- Chronic kidney disease
- Recreational drug abuse
- Chronic high stress levels

The recognition and management of these risk factors is the key to decreasing the risk of a heart attack.

The probability of a Heart attack can be determined by a Cardiac Risk Score calculated by your family doctor. This takes into consideration sex, age, blood pressure, the presence of diabetes, lipid levels and smoking. Knowledge of the cardiac risk score can assist in taking the necessary preventive measures to avoid a heart attack.

Heart Failure

Heart Failure occurs when the heart muscle is too weak to pump blood through the body effectively. This results in shortness of breath, tiredness and swelling of the legs and ankles.

The causes of heart failure include:

- Coronary heart disease (blockage of blood vessels)
- Long standing high blood pressure
- Cardiomyopathy (weakness of heart muscle)
- Diabetes
- Heart valve disease.
- Thyroid disease

The management of heart failure includes the treatment of the underlying cause, medications, and lifestyle modification.

Strokes

Around 6 million people died of strokes in 2011, worldwide.

A stroke occurs when blood supply to the Brain is suddenly interrupted.

This may be due to blockage by a clot or bleed.

Causes of Stroke include:

- High blood pressure
- Diabetes
- Smoking
- High cholesterol
- Heart disease

The management of Stroke includes the treatment of the underlying cause, physical and psychological rehabilitation.

Diabetes

Around 350 million people worldwide live with Diabetes. Complications from Diabetes lead to around 4 million deaths per year.

Diabetes (high blood sugar) occurs when inadequate amounts of Insulin are produced, or cells do not respond to the insulin which is produced.

Normal blood sugar is a fasting blood sugar of less than 5.5 mmol/l or less than 8 mmol/l, done 2 hours after a meal.

Long term control of Diabetes, is assessed by a test annotated HBAIC. The normal reading for this test is below 6.0 mmol/l. However a level of less than 7.0 mmol/l is regarded as acceptable control. In patients who suffer from Diabetes, the test is usually done every 6 months.

Types of Diabetes described are:

- Type 1 Diabetes—resulting from the body's failure to produce Insulin
- Type 2 Diabetes—resulting from cells failing to utilize Insulin properly (Insulin Resistance)
- Gestational Diabetes—Diabetes in pregnant women who have previously not suffered from Diabetes

Long term complications of Diabetes include:

- Kidney disease
- Eye disease
- Disease of blood vessels
- Disease of the nervous system
- Skin disease

The management of Diabetes and it's complications includes:

- Dietary control. Your doctor or a dietician will assist in formulating a diet plan.
- Exercise
- Not smoking
- Not overusing alcohol
- Oral medications and injections
- Home monitoring of blood sugar
- Regular check-ups with your doctor (usually 3-6 monthly) to assess control and monitor for complications.

Exercise and weight control can sometimes result in reducing or ceasing medication for Diabetes.

Kidney Disease

Around 1 million people per year die of kidney diseases worldwide.

The common causes of Chronic Kidney Disease include:

- High blood pressure

- Diabetes
- Infection
- Long term use of painkillers and anti-inflammatory medications
- Hardening of the arteries (atherosclerosis)
- Polycystic kidney disease (a genetic condition in which normal kidney tissue is replaced by multiple cysts).
- Obstruction of urine flow by Kidney Stones, an enlarged Prostate or Cancer

The prevention of Kidney disease may be achieved by:

- Regular checks to monitor for High blood pressure and Diabetes
- Drinking adequate fluids
- Not smoking
- Not overusing alcohol
- Exercising regularly
- Keeping your doctor informed of all medications you take, including medications consumed without prescription and "natural" remedies. There are a variety of medications which have potential to cause kidney damage.

Chronic Lung Diseases

Around 64 million people worldwide suffer from chronic lung diseases.

These diseases account for around 3 million deaths per year.

Chronic obstructive pulmonary disease (COPD) includes Emphysema and Recurrent/Chronic Bronchitis.

Causes of chronic lung diseases include:

- Smoking
- Exposure to Occupational Irritants
- Air pollution
- Genetics
- Recurrent Chest Infections

Chronic lung diseases can be prevented or alleviated by;

- Stopping smoking
- Prevent /reduce industry pollutant exposure with the wearing of protective equipment, and dust/irritant control measures
- Reduce air pollution. This measure is usually mediated through Government legislation and surveillance.

Depression

In 2012 the World Health Organisation estimate for sufferers of Depression worldwide was 350 million people. Of these, less than fifty percent of patients had access to treatment (in some cases as little as five percent had access). Depression sadly has far reaching consequences for both the sufferer and the extended family. It affects both physical and mental health. As there is a serious risk of self-harm and suicide, the sufferer should be monitored closely, and timely management be effected to prevent disastrous consequences.

There are variants of Depression. These include:

- Major depressive disorder

This type of depression is caused by chemical changes in the brain. It is often genetic. Adverse life events increase the chance of developing symptoms

- Psychotic depression.

This disorder is primarily genetic. It may also occur as a phase in bipolar mood disorder, and with use of recreational drugs such as cannabis or amphetamines. Symptoms of the disorder include delusions (false beliefs), hallucinations (seeing, hearing, feeling, smelling or tasting something which is not really present)

- Bipolar mood disorder

This condition presents as periods of elevated, irritable mood alternating with periods of depression.-Other signs include flights of ideas, pressured speech, antisocial and irresponsible behaviour, and decreased need for sleep

- Mixed anxiety and depression
- Dysthymia (milder form of chronic depression)
- Depression related to medical conditions, for example, thyroid disorder
- Reactive depression (due to life stresses, grief or loss)

Management of Depression

These include:

- Management by your treating doctor with counselling and medication if indicated.
- Psychiatric and Psychological management
- Hospital management.
- Family and other social support
- Support organizations, of which there are many. Your family doctor can assist in referring you to one of these organisations.

The Kessler psychological distress scale (K 10 questionnaire) is a simple tool to measure psychological distress. An abnormal score may help diagnose Depression and Anxiety. If you note that you regularly experience one or more of the following, it is advised that you seek medical attention:

- You feel depressed
- You feel anxious and nervous
- You feel chronically tired, and that everything is an effort
- You feel hopeless
- You feel so sad that nothing cheers you up
- You feel worthless
- You feel life is not worth living, or have contemplated suicide

Suicide

Sadly over 1 million lives a year are lost due to Suicide worldwide. This number surpasses deaths from any cancer, except Lung cancer, and any infectious disease except HIV/AIDS and Tuberculosis.

Causal factors in Suicide include:

- Difficulties with interpersonal relationships
- Financial difficulties
- Mental Illness such as depression, schizophrenia, bipolar mood disorder, alcoholism
- Drug Abuse
- Unemployment
- Homelessness
- War
- Genetics
- Gambling debts

Of concern is the fact that suicide is the leading cause of death in young people. The prevention of suicide requires the proactive involvement of health care providers, family and friends. Your family doctor will be able to source one or more support organisations to assist you. In the event of a crisis which leads to suicidal ideation, you are urged to call a suicide helpline available in the region in which you live.

Dementia

Dementia, of which Alzheimer's disease is the commonest type, is a progressive and eventual fatal disease affecting the brain. It impairs thinking, memory, personality, and social skills. Over 36 million people worldwide live with Dementia. In developed countries it is fast overtaking other conditions in being one of the leading causes of death.

Causes of Dementia include:

- Degeneration of brain cells without a known cause
- Conditions affecting blood vessels, and nerve disorders

- Parkinson's disease
- Infections, example Syphilis and HIV/Aids

Management of Dementia include:

- General Medical management, including drug therapy
- Psychiatric and Psychological management.-
- Support measures by Family, Friends and Support Groups

A questionnaire entitled MMSE (mini-mental state examination), may be administered by your treating doctor to screen for Dementia. Further assessment is advised if you, your family or friends have concerns with regards to your:

- Memory
- Orientation to time, place, location
- Behavioural and personality changes
- Loss of social skills

Cancer

Cancers of all types account for around fifteen percent of deaths worldwide annually. Around seventy percent of deaths from Cancer occur in middle and low income countries. Lifestyle factors, namely, smoking, alcohol abuse, obesity, inadequate consumption of vegetable and fruit, and lack of exercise, are implicated in thirty percent of cases of Cancer. Also implicated are some viral infections, such as Hepatitis B and C, and Human papilloma virus (HPV).

The reduction of Cancer risk includes avoiding the stated risk factors, vaccination against Hepatitis B and HPV, controlling occupational hazards and reducing exposure to sunlight.

Skin Cancer

Skin cancers are a particular concern in people with fair skin. The risk for skin cancer is increased by prolonged exposure to sunlight and other sources of radiation. Malignant melanoma kills over 70,000 people a year worldwide, especially in developed countries.

Major types of Skin Cancer are:

1. Melanoma
2. Squamous cell cancer
3. Basal cell cancer

Causes of Skin cancer include:

1. Over exposure to sunlight and other radiation.
2. Heredity
3. Smoking
4. Chronic non-healing wounds
5. Human Papilloma Virus (HPV) in some forms of skin cancer

Prevention of Skin Cancer includes:

1. Regular skin checks
2. Avoid over exposure to ultraviolet radiation especially during peak ultraviolet radiation times of the day when sunlight is at it's strongest (from around 10.00 am till 3.00 pm).
3. Avoid smoking
4. Wear sun protective clothing and apply sunscreen preparations
5. Do not expose yourself to solarium experiences.

Lung Cancer

Lung cancer is the leading type of Cancer causing death worldwide. The disease accounts for around 2 million deaths per year worldwide.

Causes of Lung Cancer include:

1. Smoking, including passive smoking
2. Air pollutants
3. Asbestos exposure
4. Some viruses

Prevention of Lung cancer can be achieved by:

- Non smoking
- Control and avoidance of respiratory irritants, such as asbestos, toxic gases.

Breast Cancer

Breast cancer causes over 500,000 deaths per year worldwide.

Causes of Breast Cancer include:

- Family history—around 25% of women with breast cancer have a family history of the condition
- Advancing age
- Prolonged use of Hormone replacement therapy
- Alcohol abuse
- Radiation

Preventative measures for breast cancer include:

- Self-examination of your breasts around once a month. Report any unusual symptoms, lumps or thickening to your doctor. It is important to note that self-examination does not guarantee the possibility of detecting a developing cancer.
- Periodic examinations by your doctor.
- Mammography screening over the age of 40 years.

Cancer of Cervix

Deaths from cervical cancer worldwide in 2011 exceeded 300,000.

Underlying risk factors associated with this cancer include exposure to human papilloma virus (HPV), multiple sexual partners, smoking and HIV infection.

Screening by Pap smear is recommended in sexually active females at intervals which may vary from 2-5 years in different countries. Your family doctor will advise you of the appropriate interval in your country.

Immunisation against HPV is now possible with the administration of a vaccine. You are advised to speak to your doctor regarding the advisability and timing with regards to vaccination. It should be noted that the vaccine available does not offer total protection.Other screening measures such as regular PAP smear is still important.

Prostate Cancer

The prostate gland is present in males only, and is situated just below the bladder.

Prostate cancer results in over 250,000 deaths per year in men worldwide.

The specific cause of this cancer is unknown.

There is an association with genetics, some infections, especially sexually transmitted infections, overuse of multivitamins and obesity

Protective factors for this cancer appear to include some vegetables, example broccoli and cauliflower, and supplements such as selenium.

Screening for Prostate Cancer may be achieved by periodic digital examination by your doctor combined with a PSA blood test. The value of Prostate screening tests is controversial, and is currently being reviewed. PSA test is however useful to monitor progress with treatment for patients who already have a prostate cancer.

Colon and Rectum Cancer

Over 600,000 people die of colorectal cancer annually worldwide.

Causes and risk factors include:

- Family history
- Polyps in the bowel
- Inflammatory bowel disease (Ulcerative colitis and Crohns disease)
- Smoking
- Alcohol abuse
- Some viruses
- Excessive red meats and processed meats

Prevention measures include:

- Non smoking
- Stool testing for blood every 2 years after the age of 50 years.
- Colonoscopy, if you at high risk or have a family history of colon cancer. It is advised that you check with your doctor regarding the appropriate time to commence colonoscopy and the time interval for further review.
- Eating a diet low in red meats and processed meat, and high in vegetables, fibre and fish
- Physical activity

Stomach Cancer

Stomach cancer kills over 750,000 people per year, worldwide.

Risk factors for Stomach Cancer include:

- Family history
- Smoking
- Alcohol abuse
- Helicobacter Infection (the same bacteria implicated in Peptic Ulcer)
- Diet rich in saturated fats, processed foods
- Obesity

Ways to reduce the risk of stomach cancer include not smoking, not abusing alcohol, consuming adequate vegetables and fruit, reducing animal fats and weight control.

HIV/AIDS

It was estimated that, in 2011, around 35 million people were infected with the HIV virus worldwide. Around 70% of cases are in Africa. Death from HIV related illness accounts for around 2 million people annually. HIV can be acquired through unsafe sex practices, infected needles, transfusion of infected blood, infected donor organs, and through transmission from an infected mother to her unborn child. The risk of contracting the disease is increased if one is exposed to multiple partners. HIV infection cannot be contracted by holding or kissing.

Present recommendations for HIV screening (blood test) is in the presence of other sexually transmitted infections, multiple partners, drug users (injections), health care workers who may be exposed and in pregnancy. In addition, some employers and insurers request HIV screening as part of the pre-employment medical or application for insurance.

Tuberculosis

In 2011 nearly 10 million people worldwide suffered from Tuberculosis. In the same year there were around 2 million deaths from the disease. Of the cases suffering from Tuberculosis, 25% are HIV positive as well. The disease is prevalent where poor socioeconomic conditions prevail.

Fortunately, the death rate has fallen by around 40% in the past 20 years. This has been due to immunisation, effective available treatment, improved nutrition and improvement in living conditions.

Diagnosis and screening of Tuberculosis is achieved by skin test, sputum examination and chest X-ray. Vaccination against Tuberculosis with a vaccine (BCG) is available in situations where the risk of exposure is significant. Your family doctor will advise you if you need to be vaccinated.

Malaria

In 2011, around 250 million people were infected with the Malaria parasite. The disease is transmitted by certain mosquitoes. Nearly 1 million people died of the disease in 2011.

Preventative measures include the wearing of protective clothing, the use of insecticides in the environment, the use of mosquito nets, avoiding outdoor exposure at dawn or dusk, and prevention with antimalarial drugs.

CHAPTER 5

Health Screening Guidelines

Health screening protocols vary between different countries and sometimes between states in the same country. They also change from time to time when new evidence becomes available. It is therefore necessary to check with your personal doctor as to the current guidelines. There are in addition controversies which exist as to the value or otherwise of some screening tests. The following should hence be viewed as a general guide to create awareness regarding measures to prevent disease. Time intervals for the different screening measures may vary depending on your age, sex, other risk factors, personal or family history, and variations in screening protocols in different countries. Your doctor will plan your personal health screen protocol.

Age and sex related guidelines for health screening in adults over 25 year of age

Men

General Physical Examination including:

- Blood Pressure
- Body Mass Index and Waist/Hip Ratio
- Blood Sugar
- Cholesterol
- Skin Check
- Prostate check—digital rectal examination and possible PSA check
- Colon Cancer Screen Stool Blood test every 2 years after the age of 50 years, and possibly colonoscopy if at high risk

- Dental Examination
- Vision check and Eye examination
- Immunization status check
- Osteoporosis screening
- Hearing test—commencing at age 65 years

Women

General Physical examination including:

- Blood Pressure
- Body Mass Index (Height and Weight)
- Blood Sugar
- Cholesterol.
- Pelvic Examination and Pap smear
- Breast examination
- Skin examination
- Mammography
- Bone mineral density
- Colon cancer screen (stool test for blood every 2 years after the age of 50 years, and colonoscopy if indicated)
- Immunization status check
- Dental examination
- Vision check and Eye examination

Prenatal screening

The following tests are advised for women who wish to conceive:

- Full blood examination
- Immunisation status for Rubella (German measles) and Chickenpox.
- Pap smear

Antenatal screening

The following tests are recommended early in pregnancy:

- Full blood Examination
- Blood group and antibodies
- Blood sugar/Glucose tolerance test (if at high risk)
- Rubella, Hepatitis B and C, Chlamydia, Gonorrhoea, Syphilis and HIV
- Urine examination
- Pap smear if overdue

During pregnancy screening with ultrasound and blood test can be done to assess risk for Down's syndrome.

Sexually Transmitted Infections (STI) Tests

Sexually transmitted infections (STIs) may occur through vaginal, anal or oral sexual contact. The main sexually transmitted infections are:

- Chlamydia
- Genital herpes
- Gonorrhoea
- Trichomonas infection
- Syphilis
- HIV/AIDS
- Hepatitis B and C
- Human papilloma virus (HPV)

The following are methods of both screening for infections with no symptoms present, and for confirming diagnosis for infections where symptoms are present.

(a) Swab test to detect Chlamydia, Gonorrhoea, Genital herpes and Trichomonas infection.
(b) Urine test to detect Chlamydia and Gonorrhoea.
(c) Blood tests to detect HIV, Hepatitis B and C, Syphilis, and Genital herpes. Blood test for Genital herpes is not always conclusive.

Screening for Chlamydia infection is recommended in all sexually active people aged 15-29 years, because of increased prevalence and risk of complications. Women with Chlamydia infection have up to 8% risk of infertility.

Men who have sex with men should be screened for Gonorrhoea, Chlamydia, Syphilis and HIV annually.

Screening for Hepatitis C should be done in individuals who use injections for recreational drug administration, and in people who are HIV positive.

STI screening in pregnant women has been noted previously. Certain types of HPV infection can cause cervical cancer in women.-Testing for the presence of HPV infection is achieved by PAP smear test. The test may also help detect abnormal cells which may alert one to the development of cervical cancer.

A vaccine is now available for immunisation against cervical cancer. It must be noted that the vaccine does not achieve total protection.

Anogenital warts are usually detected by your doctor at a physical examination.

Neonatal screening

Soon after birth, screening with blood tests for various congenital conditions and a hearing test can be conducted.

Occupational Health Screening

There are specific risks related to particular job descriptions which need special attention. For job descriptions which may carry a higher than usual risk of injury or death a pre-employment medical may need to be conducted on the prospective worker. In some instances, for example, the coal industry, the medical is repeated at periodic intervals (between 1-5 years).

- Audiometry (Hearing test)

Initial and periodic hearing tests form an important aspect of health surveillance in industry prone to high levels of noise. In such instances adherence to hearing protocols is established. These include wearing hearing protective aids, and minimising prolonged exposure to machinery noise.

- Spirometry (Breathing test)

Lung function testing at intervals, in industries where exposure to irritants (example asbestos, coal dust, chemicals) to the lungs is significant, helps monitor and limit damage to optimum lung function and raises awareness to possible underlying industrial diseases.

- Sleep disorder screening

Sleep apnoea (episodes of ceasing breathing) can cause daytime sleeping, accidents, reduced productivity, and interpersonal relationship problems. The consequences are worse for workers involved in safety critical work, for example, commercial drivers, train drivers and operators of heavy equipment. This condition needs to be diagnosed timeously and managed appropriately. The Epworth Sleepiness Scale or the Berlin Questionnaire are tools to help diagnose sleep disorders. If a sleep disorder is suspected, a sleep study (polysomnography) may be performed by a Specialist to confirm a sleep disorder.

- Musculoskeletal Assessment

Specific examinations need to be conducted to test back strength and flexibility, knee problems, and hand strength for those whose occupations which involve heavy manual lifting, repeated bending or twisting activities, and working in confined spaces. The examination is usually conducted by an Occupational health doctor or Occupational therapist.

- Cardiovascular Risk Assessment

In safety critical job descriptions (for example, machine operators, train and commercial drivers), it is sometimes requested that an assessment be conducted to assess the risk of a heart attack or stroke while working. The tests include an ECG, cholesterol/lipids and blood sugar. In addition blood pressure reading, smoking status, age and sex are considered. All of these are collated and the risk calculated. If the risk is assessed to be high referral to a heart specialist is arranged for further assessment.

CHAPTER 6

Leading causes of Death

The causes of death in developed and developing countries are reviewed. One is immediately struck by the wide differences between the groups. The causes in developed countries are often linked to lifestyle issues. Those in developing countries are sadly associated with poor socioeconomic circumstances.

Leading Causes of Preventable Death Worldwide (2011):

Rank

1. High Blood Pressure
2. Smoking
3. High Cholesterol
4. Malnutrition
5. Sexually Transmitted Diseases
6. Poor Diet
7. Obesity
8. Physical Inactivity
9. Alcohol consumption
10. Unsafe water and poor sanitation

Most Common Causes of Death Worldwide (2011):

Rank

1. Heart Attacks
2. Strokes
3. Respiratory Infections
4. Chronic Lung diseases.
5. Gastroenteritis
6. HIV/Aids
7. Lung and Trachea Cancer
8. Tuberculosis
9. Diabetes
10. Accidental
11. Malaria
12. Childhood diseases
13. Heart Failure
14. Self-Inflicted (Suicide)
15. Stomach Cancer
16. Liver Cirrhosis
17. Kidney Disease
18. Colon and Rectum Cancer
19. Liver Cancer
20. Measles

Leading Causes of Death for High Income Countries (2011):

Rank

1. Heart attacks
2. Stroke
3. Lung Cancer and other Respiratory Cancers.
4. Alzheimer's Disease and other Dementias
5. Chest Infections
6. Chronic Lung diseases
7. Colon and Rectum Cancers
8. Diabetes
9. Other Heart diseases (apart from Heart attacks)
10. Breast Cancer

It is evident that many of the listed causes of death in developed countries are lifestyle related (smoking, alcohol abuse, unhealthy diet, lack of exercise). There is opportunity for health care providers to engage in health education and promotion. However time constraints sometimes pose a challenge to achieving this all the time.

Leading Causes of Death in Low Income Countries (2011)

RANK

1. Chest infections
2. Diarrhoeal diseases
3. HIV/Aids
4. Heart attacks
5. Malaria
6. Strokes
7. Tuberculosis
8. Infant prematurity
9. Infant birth trauma and respiratory distress
10. Infections in infancy

The difficult solution to the health crises in developing countries is intrinsically linked to poverty, lack of infrastructure due to inadequate financial resources, lack of education and political stability. Unfortunately the road to resolving the issues is complex and will need much commitment from various parties. This will take some time to accomplish. Sadly many lives would have been lost in the in the process.

CHAPTER 7

Life Expectancy

Countries with Highest Life Expectancy (2011)

Life expectancy in the following countries ranged between 80-84 years.

The countries in alphabetical order:

Australia	Italy
Austria	Japan
Andorra	Jersey
Anguilla	Lichtenstein
Bermuda	Macau
Canada	Monaco
Cayman Islands	Netherlands
France	New Zealand
Germany	Norway
Guernsey	San Marino
Hong Kong	Singapore
Iceland	Spain
Ireland	Sweden
Isle of Man	Switzerland
Israel	United Kingdom

Countries with Lowest Life Expectancy (2011)

Life expectancy in these countries ranged between 49 years to 58 years.

The countries in alphabetical order are:

Afghanistan	Mali
Angola	Mozambique
Botswana	Namibia
Burkino Faso	Niger
Cameroon	Nigeria
Central African Republic	Republic of Congo
Chad	Rwanda
Cote d'Ivore	Sierra Leone
Democratic Republic of Congo	Somalia
Ethiopia	South Africa
Gabon	Swaziland
Guinea Bissau	Tanzania
Lesotho	Uganda
Liberia	Zambia
Malawi	Zimbabwe

Life Expectancy in relation to different Continents (2011):

Continent	Range
Africa	38 years (Continent lowest) to 62 years (Continent highest).
Asia	56 years (Laos) to 82 years (Japan)
North America	61 years (Haiti) to 81 years (Canada)
South America	66 years (Guyana) to 78 years (Costa Rica).
Oceania	64 years (Vanuatu) to 83 years (Australia).
Europe	74 years (previous Eastern Europe) to 82 years (previous Western Europe)

Of note is that Haiti was ranked among the lowest for life expectancy, compared to the United States of America which was ranked among the highest, although these countries are geographically so close to each other.

It is noted that apart from Afghanistan, all the other poorest countries are in Africa. Average life expectancy in Africa was around 15 years lower than the rest of the world population combined.

South Africa has a mixture of developed communities, living side by side with communities living in standards comparable to developing countries. It is expected that life expectancy in people of Caucasian descent will parallel that of other developed countries, and that of indigenous people would be similar to that in developing countries. Unfortunately the previous legacy of apartheid deprived the indigenous community of the same level of social benefits and health care enjoyed by people of Caucasian descent.

In the United States of America, people of Caucasian origin lived on average, 7 years longer than African-Americans (2012).

In Australia, life expectancy in the Caucasian population is around 15 years higher than the Indigenous Aborigine population (2011). Sadly, this represents the worst difference in life expectancy between citizens in any one country. Complex socio-political factors are implicated in the existence of this situation.

In New Zealand, life expectancy in Caucasians is 8-9 years higher than the Maori population (2011).

Similar discrepancies, between the rich and the poor are being noted in countries with emerging economies, such as China and India.

Chapter 8

Worldwide Wealth and Poverty

Diseases and premature death correlate closely with socioeconomic circumstances prevailing in a particular country.

World's richest and poorest countries

The following is a listing of the world's richest and poorest countries. The data is estimated by Gross domestic product (GDP) per capita purchasing power. Figures are displayed in US dollars earned per household/ per annum. The countries are listed in alphabetical order.

Wealthiest countries (2012):	Poorest Countries (2012):
Income exceeded U$40,000 pa	Income below U$2000 pa
Australia	Afghanistan
Austria	Benin
Belgium	Burkino Faso
Brunei	Burundi
Canada	Central African Republic
Denmark	Comores
Finland	Democratic Republic of Congo
France	Eritrea
Germany	Ethiopia
Hong Kong	Guinea
Iceland	Guinea Basso
Ireland	Haiti
Japan	Liberia

Kuwait
Luxembourg
Netherland
Norway
Qatar
Singapore
Sweden
Switzerland
Taiwan
United Arab Emirates
United Kingdom
United States of America

Madagascar
Malawi
Mali
Mozambique
Myanmar
Nepal
Niger
Rwanda
Sierra Leone
Togo
Uganda
Zimbabwe

It is noted that apart from Afghanistan, Haiti, Nepal and Myanmar, the rest of the countries with lowest incomes are in Africa.

A variety of socioeconomic and political factors combine to account for this human tragedy. Details relating to these factors fall outside the scope of this handbook.

CHAPTER 9

Conclusion

It is hoped that the basic insights this manual has explored will serve to stimulate interest in the topics covered. In a busy world, with the many pressures of daily living, it is easy to neglect the important issue of our personal health care. Time can slip past while hidden health problems take their toll unnoticed. Many illnesses remain asymptomatic for some time before they manifest to an extent that we become aware of their existence.-Studies have demonstrated that regular health checks substantially reduce (up to 30%) both morbidity and mortality associated with illnesses.

There is an obvious correlation between the availability of material resources, political stability, socioeconomic development and education on the one hand, and health status on the other. We yearn for the day when all of humanity will share the same level of physical and mental wellbeing. It is heartening to know that much is already being done by governments, non-government organisations and individuals to alleviate many health and other socioeconomic crises in disadvantaged communities in developing countries.

We are encouraged to:

1. Cherish the One Life we will have in this world.
2. Care for the One Body we have been endowed with.
3. Enjoy the privilege of experiencing life in all it's fullness.
4. Lend a helping hand wherever possible, to influence and uplift the life of our fellow human beings.

Sources used in the Preparation of this Book

1. World Health Organisation
    . Data and Statistics (2012)
    http://www.who.int/topics/statistics

2. NHS (United Kingdom)
    . Data Files (2012)
    http://www.nhs.uk/nacs/

3. Centers for Disease Control and Prevention (United States of America)
    . Malaria (2013)
    http://www.cdc.gov

4. Mayo Clinic (United States of America)
    . Diseases and Conditions
    http://www.mayoclinic.com/health/Diseasesindex

5. Royal Australian College of General Practice
    . Guidelines for preventative activities in General Practice, 8th Edition
    http://www.racgp.org.au/

6. Harvard School of Public Health (United States of America)
    . Cancer Resources Library
    http://www.harvard.edu/resources

7. Stanford University (United States of America)
    . Environmental Health and Safety
    http://www.stanford.edu/dept/EHS

8. American Cancer Society
    . Learn about Cancer
    http://www.cancer.org/

9. Australian Heart Foundation
    . Clinical Information
    http://www.heartfoundation.org.au/information-for-professionals

10. Cancer Council, New South Wales, Australia
    . Understanding Cancer
    http://www.cancercouncil.com.au

11. United States National Institute of Health
    http://www.nlm.nih.gov/hinfo

12. Aids Foundation of South Africa
    . Aids Facts and Myths
    http://www.southafrica.info/about/health/aids-prevention

13. British Nutrition Foundation
    . A Healthy Diet
    http://www.nutrition.org.uk

14. Tobacco in Australia
    . Smoking trends, health effects and smoking cessation
    http://www.tobaccoinaustralia.org

15. Alzheimer's Society (United Kingdom)
    . Living with Dementia
    http://www.alzheimers.org.uk

16. Black Dog Institute, Australia
    . The Psychological Toolkit
    http://www.blackdoginstitute.org.au

17. International Monetary Fund
    . Data and Statistics
    http://www.imf.org/external/index

18. Global Finance
    . World's Richest and Poorest Countries in 2013 (Pasquali and Aridas)
    http://www.gfmag.com/archives/2013

19. World Bank
    . Data and Statistics (2013)
    http://www.data.worldbank.org

20. New Zealand Government Statistics (2013)
    . Health and Life Expectancy
    http://www.stats.gov.nz

21. University of Maryland, Medical Centre, United States of America
    . Health information
    http://umms.org

22. Medical Journal of Australia, August 2007.
    Spirituality, Religion and Health, by Williams and Sternthal

PERSONAL HEALTH RECORD

Summary:

1. Medical History—Past and Present medical conditions
2. Allergies
3. Smoking status
4. Alcohol consumption
5. Immunisation schedule
6. Progress Health Record

Past Significant Medical Conditions	Date of occurrence	Date ceased

Additional:

Present Medical Conditions	Date of commencement

Additional:

Medication List

Additional:

Allergies/Medication Intolerance

Additional:

Smoking status:

Smoker: Number of cigarettes per day:

Never a smoker:

Former smoker: Date of quitting:

Alcohol Consumption: Standard drinks per week:

Immunisation Record

Immunisation	Date				

Clinical measurements and Investigations

It is suggested that your adult health record is commenced by 25 years of age. Your family doctor will advise you of the appropriate timeframe to commence each test and the recommended intervals between tests.

Men and Women

	Year				
	20	20	20	20	20 . . . .
Blood Pressure					
Height/Weight/Body mass index					
Blood Sugar					
Cholesterol/Lipids					
Other pathology Tests					

X-ray/Scan results

Date	Findings

Skin examination findings

Date	Findings

Colon cancer stool test/ Colonoscopy findings

Date	Findings

Dental Examination/procedures

Date	Procedures

Vision check/Eye examination Findings

Date	Findings

Dr. Yan Perumal

Hearing Test/Audiometry

Date	Findings

Bone density

Date	Result

Tests for Men Only

Prostate

Digital examination findings

Date	Findings

PSA (blood test) result

Date	Result

Tests for Women Only

PAP smear result

Date	Result

Breast examination /Mammogram findings

Date	Findings

Specialist Reports

Date	Report

INDEX

www.ingramcontent.com/pod-product-compliance
Lightning Source LLC
Chambersburg PA
CBHW030518290526
45786CB00004B/1517